SIMPLE WAY TO IMPROVE EYESIGHT INSTANTLY!

Natural Vision Improvement for Clear, Close, Distant Vision & Astigmatism Removal

DR. HELEN PAUL

Table of Contents

CHAPTER ONE

What Is Astigmatism?

Astigmatism is a condition where your eye isn't totally adjusted. Practically we all have it somewhat.

Preferably, an eyeball is molded like an impeccably round ball. Light comes into it and twists equally, which gives you an unmistakable view. In any case, if your eye is formed increasingly like a football, light gets twisted more one way than another. That implies just piece of an item is in center. Things a good ways off may look hazy and wavy.

It's entirely expected to have astigmatism alongside partial blindness (nearsightedness) or farsightedness (hyperopia). These three conditions are called refractive blunders since they include how your eyes twist (refract) light.

Astigmatism is genuinely simple for an eye specialist to fix with glasses, contacts, or medical procedure.

Astigmatism is a typical vision condition that causes obscured vision. It happens when the cornea (the unmistakable title page of the eye) is sporadically formed or now and then due to the ebb and flow of the focal point inside the eye.

Side effects of astigmatism may include:

Hazy or twisted vision

Eye fatigue

Cerebral pains

Issue seeing around evening time.

Astigmatism Causes

The vast majorities are brought into the world with it; however specialists don't have a clue why. You can likewise get it after eye damage, an eye sickness, or medical procedure.

Once in a while, a condition called keratoconus can cause astigmatism by making the unmistakable front piece of your eye (your cornea) more slender and more cone-formed. You'll most likely need contacts (yet not glasses) to see unmistakably.

You can't get astigmatism from perusing in low light or sitting excessively near the TV.

Astigmatism Diagnosis

Astigmatism side effects please gradually. Go to an eye specialist on the off chance that you see changes in your vision. You'll require a total eye test. Your primary care physician will test the sharpness of your vision by requesting that you read an eye diagram. They'll likewise utilize apparatuses to gauge your vision, including:

Phoropter. You glance through a progression of focal points to locate the ones that give you the most clear vision.

Keratometer/topographer. This machine utilizes a hover of light to quantify the bend of your cornea.

Autorefractor. This gadget sparkles light into your eye and measures how it changes as it bobs off the back. This gives your primary care physician a thought of which focal points you need.

CHAPTER TWO

Your solution will have a few letters and numbers. OD implies oculus dexter, your correct eye, and OS is oculus evil, your left eye. OU implies oculus uterque, or the two eyes.

The numbers are estimations called diopters.

The principal number is for something many refer to as circular remedy. In the event that it has a short sign, you're myopic. In the event that there's an or more sign, you're farsighted. A higher number methods blurrier vision.

The subsequent numbers are your tube shaped amendment. This is the manner by which solid your astigmatism is.

The third one is the hub, the area of the astigmatism on your cornea.

For instance, a remedy of "OD - 1.00 x - 2.00 x 155" signifies your correct eye has 1 diopter of myopia and 2 diopters of astigmatism at 155 degrees on your cornea.

Glasses or contacts can address practically all instances of astigmatism. Be that as it may, in the event that you have just a slight astigmatism and no other vision issues, you may not require them.

There are two medicines for the basic degrees of astigmatism:

Restorative focal points. That implies glasses or contacts. On the off chance that you have astigmatism, your PCP will most likely endorse an extraordinary kind of delicate contact focal points called toric focal points. They can twist light more one way than the other. On the off chance that your case is increasingly extreme, you may get gas-porous inflexible contact focal points for a methodology called orthokeratology. You wear the focal points while you rest, what's more, they reshape your cornea. You'll have to continue wearing the focal points to hold this new shape, yet you won't need to wear them as frequently.

Refractive medical procedure. Laser medical procedure likewise changes the state of your cornea. Sorts of refractive medical procedure incorporate LASIK and PRK. You'll have to have generally sound eyes with no retina issues or corneal scars.

Unpredictable astigmatism is far less normal and is connected to issues with your cornea, the front piece of the eye. Keratoconus is one model.

Numerous babies are brought into the world with astigmatism, and it frequently leaves before their first birthday celebration.

Since kids typically can't tell that there's an issue with their vision, they need ordinary eye tests beginning around a half year of age. A kid with an untreated vision condition may make some hard memories at school, and this could prompt an off base learning issue conclusion.

Finding

Astigmatism is analyzed by an eye test. A total eye test includes a progression of tests to check your eye wellbeing and a refraction, which decides how your eyes twist light. Your eye specialist may utilize different instruments, point brilliant lights straightforwardly at your eyes and request that you glance through a few focal points. Your primary care physician utilizes these tests to inspect various parts of your eyes and vision and to decide the medicine expected to give clear vision eyeglasses or contact focal points.

CHAPTER THREE

The objective of treating astigmatism is to improve vision clearness and eye comfort. Medicines are remedial focal points or refractive medical procedure.

Remedial focal points

Wearing remedial focal points treats astigmatism by checking uneven bends of your cornea and focal point.

Sorts of restorative focal points include:

Eyeglasses. Eyeglasses are made with focal points that help make up for the uneven state of your eye. The focal points make the light twist into your eye appropriately. Eyeglasses can likewise address for other refractive mistakes, for example, astigmatism or farsightedness.

Contact focal points. Like eyeglasses, contact focal points can address most astigmatism. They are accessible in an assortment of types and styles, including expendable delicate; expanded wear; inflexible, gas porous; and bifocal.

Contact focal points are likewise utilized in a method called orthokeratology. In orthokeratology, you wear unbending contact focal points during the night while dozing until the arch of your eye levels out. At that point you wear the focal points less oftentimes to keep up the new shape. In the event that you stop this treatment, your eyes come back to their previous shape and refractive blunder.

Wearing contact focal points for broadened timeframes expands the danger of contamination in the eye.

Get some information about the advantages and disadvantages and dangers of contact focal points and what may be best for you.

Refractive medical procedure improves vision and lessens the requirement for eyeglasses or contact focal points. Your eye specialist utilizes a laser pillar to reshape the bends of the cornea, which revises the refractive blunder. Prior to medical procedure, specialists will assess you and decide whether you're a contender for refractive medical procedure.

Kinds of refractive medical procedure for astigmatism include:

Laser-aided situ keratomileusis (LASIK). With this technique, your eye specialist makes a slim, pivoted fold in your cornea. The individual in question uses an excimer laser to shape the state of the cornea and afterward repositions the fold.

Laser-helped subepithelial keratectomy (LASEK). Rather than making a fold in the cornea, the specialist slackens the cornea's meager defensive spread (epithelium) with an uncommon liquor. The person in question uses an excimer laser to change the arch of the cornea and afterward repositions the relaxed epithelium.

Photorefractive keratectomy (PRK). This methodology is like

LASEK, aside from the specialist expels the epithelium. It will develop back normally, fitting in with your cornea's new shape. You may need to wear a wrap contact focal point for a couple of days after medical procedure.

Epi-LASIK. This is a variety of LASEK. Your primary care physician utilizes an uncommon motorized gruff cutting edge — rather than the liquor — to isolate a meager sheet of epithelium. The individual in question at that point utilizes an excimer laser to reshape the cornea and repositions the epithelium.

Little cut lenticule extraction (SMILE). This more up to date kind of refractive medical procedure reshapes the cornea by utilizing a laser to make a focal point molded piece of tissue (lenticule) underneath the cornea surface. The lenticule is then expelled through a little entry point. Until further notice, the SMILE methodology is endorsed for treating gentle astigmatism.

Different sorts of refractive medical procedures incorporate clear focal point extraction and implantable contact focal points. There is nobody best strategy for refractive medical procedure and the choice should just be made after a total assessment and careful discourse with your specialist.

A portion of the potential difficulties that can happen after refractive medical procedure include:

Undercorrection or overcorrection of your underlying issue

Visual reactions, for example, a corona or starburst showing up around lights

Dry eye

Disease

Corneal scarring

Once in a while, vision misfortune

Talk about the potential dangers and advantages of these strategies with your eye specialist.

Planning for your arrangement

You may experience three sorts of pros as you look for help for different eye conditions:

Ophthalmologist. An ophthalmologist is an eye authority with a specialist of medication (M.D.) or a specialist of osteopathy (D.O.) degree who gives full eye care. This consideration incorporates performing total eye assessments, recommending remedial focal points, diagnosing and treating normal and complex eye issue, and performing eye medical procedure when it's essential.

Optometrist. An optometrist has a specialist of optometry (O.D.) degree. Optometrists are prepared to give eye wellbeing assessments, endorse restorative focal points, and analyze and treat some eye conditions.

Optician. An optician is a master who assists fit with peopling for eyeglasses following solutions from ophthalmologists and optometrists. A few states expect opticians to be authorized. Opticians are not prepared to analyze or treat eye illness.

Regardless of which sort of eye expert you pick, here's some data

to assist you with preparing for
your arrangement.

CHAPTER FOUR

What you can do?

Rundown any manifestations you're encountering, including any that may appear to be random to the purpose behind which you booked the arrangement.

Rundown key individual data, including any significant anxieties or late life changes.

Make a rundown everything being equal, nutrients or enhancements that you're taking, including portions.

Rundown inquiries to pose to your primary care physician.

Astigmatism (uh-STIG-muh-tiz-um) is a typical and for the most part treatable blemish in the ebb and flow of your eye that causes obscured remove and close to vision.

Astigmatism happens when either the front surface of your eye (cornea) or the focal point, inside your eye, has confused bends. Rather than having one bend like a round ball, the surface is egg formed. This causes obscured vision at all separations.

Astigmatism is regularly present during childbirth and may happen in mix with myopia or farsightedness. Regularly it's not articulated enough to require restorative activity. At the point when it is, your treatment choices are remedial focal points or medical procedure.

Signs and indications of astigmatism may include:

Obscured or misshaped vision

Eye fatigue or uneasiness

Cerebral pains

Trouble with night vision

Squinting

See an eye specialist if your eye side effects cheapen your happiness regarding exercises or meddle with your capacity to perform regular errands. An eye specialist can decide if you have astigmatism and, assuming this is the case, to what degree. The individual in question would then be able to inform you with respect to your choices to address your vision.

Kids may not understand their vision is hazy, so they should be screened for eye infection and have their vision tried by a pediatrician, an ophthalmologist, an optometrist or another prepared screener at the accompanying ages and interims.

During the infant time frame

At well-kid visits until school age

During school years, each one to two years at well-kid visits, at the eye specialist, or through school or open screenings

Causes

Disentangled life structures of the eye

Astigmatism

Your eye has two structures with bended surfaces that curve (refract) light onto the retina, which makes the pictures:

The cornea, the reasonable front surface of your eye alongside the tear film

The focal point, a reasonable structure inside your eye that changes shape to help center around close to objects

In an impeccably formed eye, every one of these components has a round ebb and flow, similar to the outside of a smooth ball. A cornea and focal point with such ebb and flow twist (refract) all approaching light similarly to make a forcefully centered picture legitimately around the retina, at the back of your eye.

CHAPTER FIVE

A refractive blunder

In the event that either your cornea or focal point is egg molded with two bungled bends, light beams aren't bowed the equivalent, which structures two unique pictures. These two pictures cover or join and result in obscured vision. Astigmatism is a kind of refractive mistake.

Astigmatism happens when your cornea or focal point is bended more steeply one way than in another. You have corneal astigmatism if your cornea has confounded bends. You have lenticular astigmatism if your focal point has confounded bends.

Either kind of astigmatism can cause obscured vision. Obscured vision may happen more one way, either on a level plane, vertically or slantingly.

Astigmatism might be available from birth, or it might create after eye damage, infection or medical procedure. Astigmatism isn't caused or aggravated by perusing in poor light, sitting excessively near the TV or squinting.

Other refractive mistakes

Astigmatism may happen in blend with other refractive mistakes, which include:

Partial blindness (nearsightedness). This happens when your cornea is bended to an extreme or your eye is longer than ordinary. Rather than being centered decisively around your retina, light is engaged before your retina, causing inaccessible items to appear to be foggy.

Farsightedness (hyperopia). This happens when your cornea is bended excessively little or your eye is shorter than typical. The impact is something contrary to partial blindness. At the point when your eye is in a casual state, light never goes to an emphasis on the back of your eye, making close by objects appear to be foggy.

Astigmatism is analyzed by an eye test. A total eye test includes a progression of tests to check your eye wellbeing and a refraction, which decides how your eyes twist light. Your eye specialist may utilize different instruments, point brilliant lights straightforwardly at your eyes and request that you glance through a few focal points. Your PCP utilizes these tests to inspect various parts of your eyes and vision and to decide the remedy expected to give clear vision eyeglasses or contact focal points.

THE END.